An Easy Way
To Understand
Fibromyalgia

Also By Brian B Jacques

His very popular Series of Mini-Health Books includes:

- An Easy Way To Understand Eczema and Psoriasis
- An Easy Way To Understand Stress and Depression
- An Easy Way To Understand Vitamins and Minerals
- An Easy Way To Understand Parasites, Worms, Candida, Constipation & Detoxing
- An Easy Way To Understand Crohn's Disease and IBD
- An Easy Way To Understand Body Building For Men And Women
- An Easy Way To Understand Alzheimer's Disease
- An Easy Way To Understand Herpes
- An Easy Way To Understand Parkinson's Disease
- An Easy Way To Understand Autism
- An Easy Way To Understand Fibromyalgia
- An Easy Way To Understand Your Body Systems
- An Easy Way To Understand Erectile Dysfunction
- An Easy Way To Understand Heart Disease, High Blood Pressure & Stroke
- An Easy Way To Understand Detoxing For Men & Women
- How To Lose Weight After 40
- How To Lose Weight And Maintain Your Ideal Weight Permanently
- Amino Acids & Enzymes—What Are They & Why Do You Need Them
- The Little A–Z Dictionary of Herbal Remedies
- The Magic Of Vitamins & Minerals
- Effective Methods To Stop Smoking
- Eat Wholefoods And Take Supplements—The Ultimate Lifestyle Guide
- Stress Busters Adult Coloring Book

All these books are available as Kindle Editions (available from the Kindle Store on Amazon.com, and other countries Amazon sites where the Kindle platform is supported.) Many of these books are also available for the Barnes and Noble "Nook". In addition, many of these titles are available as print editions from the Amazon website.

An Easy Way
To Understand
Fibromyalgia

Brian B Jacques

Wisdom For Life Media

Publisher: Wisdom For Life Media (www.wisdomforlifemedia.com)

While they have made every effort to verify the information provided in this publication, neither the author nor the publisher assumes any responsibility for errors in, omissions from, or different interpretation of the subject matter.

The information herein may be subject to varying laws, regulations, and practices in different areas, states and countries. The purchaser or reader assumes all responsibility for use of the information.

All information included within this book is for educational purposes only. The author and publishers do not attempt to diagnose or treat any medical conditions, be it to do with health, diet or exercise.

If you consider that you have any kind of medical condition, then, you should consult a qualified medical practitioner or doctor or qualified naturopathic doctor before starting any herbal, vitamin and/or mineral program or supplement regime, exercise or health training program or diet suggested in this book.

This book is not intended for anyone under the age of 18 years, nor is it intended for breast feeding or pregnant women, underweight people or anyone with eating disorders or a health condition that requires special diets or medical treatment.

The author and publishers disclaim any liability for any loss however caused by anyone using the information contained in this book.

ISBN - 13: 978-1546798552

ISBN - 10: 1546798552

Published in The United States of America.

"Education is the kindling of a flame, not the filling of a vessel." —Socrates

Contents

Acknowledgment

To the many people I have come into contact with throughout my life, whose belief in me has made everything possible and worthwhile.

Chapter 1. Symptoms

The cause of fibromyalgia is unknown, there is no cure and in addition, it is not well understood. Therefore, having a physician do an evaluation of the symptoms, and provide a definite diagnosis of a fibromyalgia condition is essential, if a treatment protocol is to be put in place for an individual, who is experiencing symptoms of fibromyalgia. This should mean that they will be able to obtain some relief from the pain and improve their quality of life.

Whilst primary symptoms of fibromyalgia are tenderness in the muscles as well as pain, other areas of the body are also affected; for example the digestive system as well as mental processing. Because there is this overlapping of symptoms a physician or patient can often refer to fibromyalgia not as a disease or illness, but as a syndrome.

I have provided some of the symptoms of fibromyalgia at the end of this chapter. They are provided for your guidance only, and if you suspect you have fibromyalgia then it is important that you get a proper diagnosis from a physician to ensure that other possible causes of your discomfort are not overlooked.

The American College of Rheumatology states that fibromyalgia affects approximately 3 to 6 million people in the United States. Roughly 20 times more women than men suffer from the syndrome.

Women between the age of 20 and 60 are at greatest risk. Therefore, if a woman is suffering from fibromyalgia it is important that she consults a gynecologist who has experience in coaching women through questions about their menstrual periods, as well as pregnancy and delivery.

It is important to understand that not all symptoms will appear equally in all individuals. Some individuals may exhibit many of the symptoms while others may only experience a few. There is some evidence to suggest that the symptoms of fibromyalgia appear after an illness or a traumatic event such as a car accident.

Fibromyalgia is evidenced by tender points—especially when pressure is applied; specific pain areas include: the neck, shoulders, between the shoulder blades, hips and areas of the spine, the back of the head, the upper back, upper chest, elbows, lower back, hips, thighs and the inner part of the knees. It mainly affects muscles and areas of attachment to the bone, however, other areas of the body can be affected too. In some ways it can feel like an individual is suffering from arthritis, but no deformity of the joints is experienced, and in most cases there is no swelling either.

Here is a list of symptoms:

- Cramps in the legs as well as muscle pain and muscle spasms
- Getting up in the morning and feeling just as tired as when you went to bed
- Insomnia
- Disturbed sleep patterns
- Pain in the muscles in specific points which have been identified in fibromyalgia sufferers
- Alpha EEG anomaly—a sleep disorder
- Muscle pain over specific trigger points identified in people with FMS
- Widespread pain
- Changes in mood
- Irritable bowel syndrome
- Regular headaches
- Pain that is widespread throughout the body
- Feelings of nausea
- Grinding of teeth
- Restless Leg Syndrome
- Acid Reflux
- GERD – Gastroesophageal Reflux
- Pain in the chest
- Tingling or numbness in the hands and feet
- Skin that is sensitive
- Dry mouth and dry eyes
- Arms and legs that feels swollen

- A sensitivity to bright lights, noises and on occasions medications
- Feelings of dizziness
- Twitching muscles
- A gain in weight
- A decline in energy in addition to moderate or severe fatigue
- Muscle stiffness after waking up or being in one position for any length of time
- A decline in concentration or memory
- Tenderness in the jaw and facial area
- Feelings of anxiety or depression
- An increased inability to perform exercise routines
- Menstrual periods that are painful
- Bladder irritation

Various factors that can aggravate fibromyalgia symptoms:

- Weather changes
- Menstrual cycle
- Allergies
- Being under stress
- Depression
- Being anxious
- Over-exerting oneself

Fibromyalgia symptoms can be worse during different periods of the day. For the majority of people the worst times are early in the morning and late in the afternoon. Hormonal fluctuations can increase the intensity of the symptoms during menstrual periods.

Although there is no cure for fibromyalgia, with the correct treatment protocols the symptoms can be reduced to a manageable level. This is the reason why it is important to get an early diagnosis of the condition so that appropriate treatments can be put in place.

Chapter 2. Causes

Researchers have been unable to determine what actually causes fibromyalgia syndrome, although several theories have been put forward.

One theory suggests that people who suffer from fibromyalgia experience a lower threshold for pain due to an increased sensitivity in the brain to pain signals. This is brought about by increased stimulation of the nerves which has the effect of causing changes in the brain resulting in increased levels of neurotransmitters.

The thinking is that the brain cells receiving the signals have somehow the ability to store a degree of memory and as a result become more sensitive, this then creates an overreaction to the stimuli. Researchers also wonder if people who suffer from fibromyalgia also had a reduced threshold to pain as a child.

What causes confusion is that there are many overlapping factors involving various body systems which could suggest that many factors could be involved.

Factors that could be involved include sleep patterns which could be one cause of the problem; an injury sustained to an area involving the upper spinal cord which could start the development of fibromyalgia; a bacterial or viral infection that may trigger symptoms; a genetic link involving abnormalities in the nervous system or possibly changes in the metabolism of the muscle structure.

Researchers have identified that hormonal changes as well as stress levels can increase levels of pain in sufferers. In addition, researchers theorize that these two factors could be one of the causes involved in changes in pain levels in the body.

Regarding a genetic link, in studies involving the family history of sufferers it was found that other family members often suffer from the same condition. This leads researchers to suggest that there is a trigger mechanism involving the factors listed above.

As there are more women than men who suffer from fibromyalgia researchers are focusing on finding a hormonal trigger that could be a cause of the syndrome.

Because fibromyalgia is such a complex syndrome that affects many thousands of people each year, in which some people have such severe symptoms that it causes them to be unable to pursue their careers, and in the case of students, it affects their ability to do well at college. It is therefore essential to get an early diagnosis and treatment protocol in place to help lessen the effects of this debilitating syndrome.

Chapter 3. Fibromyalgia verses Polymyalgia

The word "myalgia" means muscle pain, and is a symptom of a variety of different conditions. Fibromyalgia and polymyalgia are categorized as two of these conditions, and although the name myalgia is involved in both of them, they are quite different conditions in their effect upon the human body.

Common symptoms of both these conditions include: depression, fatigue, stiffness when waking up in the morning, and is present in more women than men. Both these conditions can prove difficult for a physician to diagnose. So now let us have a look at the differences.

As mentioned previously, fibromyalgia is often referred to as a syndrome—in fact a chronic illness. Every part of the body can suffer where fibrous tissue is involved; this includes ligaments and tendons, and the effect does not just involve muscle pain. Spasms of the muscles and a muscle burning sensation are often associated with someone who has a fibromyalgia condition.

A fibromyalgia condition does not involve an inflammatory condition as is the case with polymyalgia, and as a result, fibromyalgia is far more difficult to provide an effective treatment for. Anyone of any age and sex can be affected with fibromyalgia.

Treatments tend to focus on drug therapy to help alleviate symptoms and provide an improved quality of life. In their search for relief from the pain, many sufferers embark on an alternative treatment regime. I have included a chapter on vitamin and herbal products later in this book.

Let us now look at polymyalgia or as it is often called polymyalgia rheumatica. This condition affects the muscle areas as well as the joints. This condition also causes inflammation whilst fibromyalgia does not. Polymyalgia mainly affects elderly people. It is very unlikely to find anyone with polymyalgia under the age of 50 years. Common factors include if you have giant cell arteritis, are a woman, and/or your ancestors came from Scandinavia or northern European countries.

Researchers are not sure of the origins of this condition although there is a genetic factor involved, especially rheumatoid arthritis or possibly environmental factors. Common symptoms include: stiffness as well as pain in the muscles of the hips, neck, shoulders, upper arms, upper thighs, as well as loss of appetite, fever, and weight loss. What is alarming is that these symptoms can appear without warning and in some cases very suddenly, possibly overnight.

Tests performed to determine a polymyalgia diagnosis include: analyzing the blood using an erythrocyte sedimentation rate and a rheumatoid factor or RF. If the diagnosis is positive chances are that later on you may develop a condition called temporal arteritis also known as giant cell arteritis. Common treatments for polymyalgia include an exercise regime, medications as well as eating a healthy diet.

It is import to understand that whilst both these conditions have similarities there are differences, in that's in fibromyalgia there is no inflammation whereas in polymyalgia there is.

Chapter 4. Research

A lot of research is underway to try and discover the causes of fibromyalgia. Here is some of the research which is being conducted by The National Institute of Arthritis and Musculoskeletal and Skin Diseases (NIAMS). The purpose of a lot of this research is not only to determine the cause of the condition, but also to identify treatment options to alleviate some of the pain.

Let me start with research into the possible relationship between hypothyroidism and fibromyalgia, as well as research into providing a better understanding of how the body deals with the processing of pain. As mentioned in a previous chapter people who suffer from fibromyalgia often have hypersensitivity to stimuli that in a non-sufferer would not cause pain. Researchers are looking for reasons why people who suffer from fibromyalgia have such sensitivity to pain. There is one theory that as more women than men suffer from fibromyalgia there could be a possible link between a female's reproductive hormones and the condition.

Taking this research a stage further will involve an examination of the role that sex hormones play in the condition and what a person's reaction to pain is. The effects of stress and other stimuli at specific times during a female's menstrual cycle will also be examined. The research will include women who have been diagnosed with fibromyalgia and those who do not have the condition.

Research is also being conducted on how a person's stress levels have an impact on how a person is able to handle physical pain. Researchers are also examining chemical reactions that happen between the endocrine and nervous systems to try and better understand the different ways in which the body responds to emotional and physical stress and whether these stress triggers can influence a reoccurrence of the combination and/or cause deterioration.

Further research is also underway to try and find a way to help fibromyalgia sufferers improve their sleep patterns. It is known that some people have difficulty sleeping even after undergoing treatment.

Family connections are also part of the research as it has been noted that fibromyalgia can occur in families. Researchers theorize that a specific gene may be responsible which may put a person more at risk of developing the condition.

Research is also being undertaken to see if there is a common link between fibromyalgia and other conditions and disorders which may be linked in families; these conditions can include such things as certain types of arthritis as well as mood swings.

The purpose of all this research is not only to identify the cause of fibromyalgia but also to develop improved treatment protocols to provide more effective relief for all the sufferers of this chronic condition worldwide.

Chapter 5. Depression

It is often the case that medical conditions occur in two's! And fibromyalgia and depression often occur together. Where fibromyalgia is involved, the persistent aches and pain which is associated with this condition often causes depression as a consequence of having to put up with the syndrome.

Fibromyalgia is not a psychological illness—it is physiological, however the condition leads many individuals who are suffering from the condition to be diagnosed with depression as well. Anxiety and depression is often caused by the stress of living with constant pain, in addition to going through the process of having an accurate diagnosis done. In many cases a person is unlikely to receive support from the medical profession, or even family and friends.

As a result of no one believing that the individual is in so much pain, the person begins to have self-doubts with the resulting feeling that it might all be in their head. This lack of support—especially from close family members, in addition to trying to cope with the debilitating symptoms of fibromyalgia, is one of the reasons why many people develop depression and as a result have to deal with this as well.

Similar symptoms occur in both fibromyalgia and depression, and as a result, it is sometimes difficult for a person to be diagnosed with one condition or the other, or indeed if they have both. As a matter of interest, depression on occasions can cause muscle aches and pains, in addition to more common symptoms such as headaches and fatigue which can make an accurate diagnosis more difficult.

Any type of illness that involves constant pain can have a depressing effect on any individual. In addition, not been able to participate in enjoyable activities which were performed before, as well as possibly needing help with daily chores which the majority of people who are not suffering from the syndrome do automatically, can lead to a feeling of anger, frustration, worthlessness and isolation.

The following is a list of some of the symptoms of depression which develop due to having fibromyalgia syndrome:

- Low energy levels
- Continual and excessive feelings of sadness or anxiety

- Having difficulty in making simple decisions and having diffi-
  culty concentrating
- Having no interest in activities that were important before in
  a person's life
- Having difficulty controlling tearful outburst
- Extreme irritability in addition to a feeling of hopelessness

To sum up, fibromyalgia and depression are often linked together. And it is reassuring to know that there are ways to relieve some
of the symptoms of both conditions. It is important for the person
who is feeling depressed to understand that they have this condition,
and it is also important that close family and friends realize what
is happening, and as result, give the person adequate support and
understanding.

Chapter 6. C-Reactive Protein (CRP) and Erythrocyte Sedimentation Rate (ESR)

Methods used to determine a possible diagnosis of fibromyalgia involve tests for C-reactive protein (CRP) and Erythrocyte Sedimentation Rate (ESR). Elevated levels of these suggest that there is inflammation somewhere in the body. So why are C-reactive protein and Erythrocyte Sedimentation Rate associated with fibromyalgia? The answer is they have a close relationship. Although the relationship is close, they are not specifically linked to fibromyalgia, as fibromyalgia is not an inflammatory condition. There are various conditions that can cause elevated CRP and ESR levels, these include:

- Infections
- Rheumatoid arthritis
- Inflammatory bowel disease (IBD)
- Cardiovascular disease
- Cancer

A plasma protein—C-reactive protein levels become elevated when there is inflammation in the body. CRP tests can be a useful indicator after a person has been diagnosed with fibromyalgia, to monitor flare ups of any disease activity in the body; in addition, they can be used to assess how effective any treatment is.

Other tests that can be performed include a physical examination where specific pressure points on the body will be pushed to determine if there is any pain in that particular area. If there is any pain in 11 out of 18 of these pressure points, the person is likely to be diagnosed with fibromyalgia, in which case, they may be referred to a rheumatologist whose speciality is muscles and joint disorders.

As there is currently no cure for fibromyalgia CRP and ESR levels where treatment is prescribed will need to be carefully monitored along with the fibromyalgia treatment. It is important to find a balance in the treatment protocols to enable the sufferer to lead as normal a daily life as possible. The main goal is always to provide relief from pain, and to help the person receive relief from any other symptoms that may be apparent as a result of this condition.

Chapter 7. Low Thyroid Levels

Low thyroid levels affect many people's everyday lives, and many people go undiagnosed. There is also a link, in that many people who suffer from fibromyalgia also have low thyroid levels. This link leads researchers to suggest there is a possible association between the two conditions.

A condition called hypothyroidism means that the person has an underactive thyroid, a symptom of which is a feeling of musculoskeletal pain and fatigue. Interestingly, these are also symptoms of fibromyalgia, or conversely what is thought of as possibly fibromyalgia could in fact be an underactive thyroid. As just stated, both conditions share many of the same symptoms leading researchers to suggest that fibromyalgia is possibly an underlying thyroid deficiency.

Performing an accurate diagnosis of hypothyroidism can sometimes prove difficult for practitioners, and as a result, it often goes untreated. As the condition does not improve many people then begin to speculate that they could possibly be developing fibromyalgia or even rheumatoid arthritis. As a result, some doctors may or may not prescribe medications that treat a thyroid deficiency, without doing further investigation to determine the true underlying cause.

However there are many enlightened doctors who now understand that fibromyalgia is just one of many symptoms associated with an underactive thyroid, and as a result, work at treating the symptoms with appropriate medications.

One study conducted by Dr. John Lowe in 1997, which is published in the Clinical Bulletin of Myofascial Therapy, determined that 64 percent of fibromyalgia patients also suffer from thyroid hormone deficiencies. This study shows that there is a definite relationship between the two conditions. The study also highlighted that there may be a link between fibromyalgia syndrome and thyroid hormone resistance syndrome which results in some people having a resistance to certain conventional thyroid medications.

As mentioned in the chapter on research much work is underway to find a possible relationship between the two conditions discussed in this chapter; the outcome of this research will play a significant role in helping develop effective treatment options. Of significance, it is known that people who suffer from fibromyalgia in most cases also have low thyroid hormone levels. Whether or not fibromyalgia and low thyroid hormone levels are linked conditions or something entirely separate as yet to be fully determined.

Chapter 8. Treatments and Medications

Various factors are involved in fibromyalgia; therefore there is a variety of treatment protocols available to deal with all these factors. Some of these factors involve stiffness in joints and muscles, feelings of nausea, headaches, as well as widespread pain and severe menstrual cramps. Treatments available include medications as well as personal options including exercise programs, treatments to restore sleep patterns and implementing a good nutrition program.

The primary goal of any treatment program is to alleviate the symptoms the patient is experiencing and improve their general quality of life. Because symptoms of fibromyalgia often affect a person's emotional, mental as well as physical health, it is important to focus on these areas so that the individual can continue to pursue their career as well as a good quality of family life.

As people who suffer from fibromyalgia are often more sensitive to medications than non-sufferers, lower dosages of medications are often recommended.

Medications can be prescribed which can help improve sleep patterns. Much work is being done by researchers in this particular area, as they feel that disturbed sleep patterns may be a trigger for the fibromyalgia disease, and it may be in some way linked to decreasing the feelings of pain and other symptoms of the disease.

Sleep Modifiers:

Taking sleep modifiers have provided short-term benefits for some individuals to restore their sleep patterns. However, doctors do not recommend this type of medication for long-term use. One of the reasons for this is that the body gets used to this type of medication and builds up a resistance against it. In addition, these types of medications are known to be addictive and as a result are used in moderation. Examples of sleep modifiers include: Eszopiclone (Lunesta), Zolpidem (Ambien), and to treat insomnia—Temazepam (Restoril) may be prescribed.

Much work is being done by researchers in the area of disturbed sleep patterns, as they feel that disturbed sleep patterns may be a trigger for fibromyalgia syndrome, and it may be in some way linked to decreasing the feelings of pain and other symptoms of the disease.

Analgesics:

Pain and stiffness can be decreased by administering analgesics such as Tylenol. However, as each individual is different and experiences different symptoms, the effectiveness of this type of medication will therefore vary.

One analgesic called Ultram has been prescribed to reduce pain. However, this medication has proved to be addictive in a similar way to opiates.

Another analgesic—Acetaminophen can be obtained as an over-the-counter (OTC) medication. The purpose is to block the pain from the body's central pathway of the nervous system. For those individuals who suffer from severe pain narcotics such as Morphine and Hydrocodone may be prescribed.

Anti-Inflammatories:

Whilst fibromyalgia is a non-inflammatory condition, anti-inflammatory medications are often prescribed to help reduce pain that is associated with tendinitis, bursitis, and/or excessive physical exertion. Examples of anti-inflammatory medications include: aspirin, ibuprofen and naproxen. Then there are Non-Steroidal Anti-Inflammatory Drugs (NSAIDS) such as Etodolac (Lodine), Nabumetone (Relafen) and Naproxyn (Anaprox). Cox-11 inhibitors such as Celebrex (Celecoxib) and the corticosteroids: Dexamethasone and Prednisone (Deltasone).

Often times NSAIDs can be combined with other medications to reduce pain.

Antidepressants:

As mentioned elsewhere in this book, people who suffer from fibromyalgia often have symptoms of depression. And whilst antidepressant medications are beneficial in treating depressive symptoms, there has been a beneficial side effect of this particular class of medications in that it is also effective in improving sleep patterns and decreasing the perception of pain. Examples of antidepressants include Duloxetine (Cymbalta) and Savella (Milnacipran).

The pain perception decrease is also being linked to a new class of anti-depressant medications called serotonin reuptake inhibitors (SSRIs). These medications regulate certain chemicals in the brain which are linked to the transmission of pain signals.

Muscle Relaxers:

these are designed to reduce pain by providing a muscle relaxing agent to the central neurological action of the muscles, but they do not reduce muscle spasms.

Some individuals have had positive results by using muscle relaxants especially at bedtime to reduce the effects of muscle pain and spasms while they sleep. It is important to understand that this type of medication should only be taken at night as it may cause drowsiness if taken during the daytime.

It is also useful to undertake an exercise program to help reduce the pain perception. In addition, if muscle relaxant medications are taken during the daytime, then it will be next to impossible to complete any exercise program. The benefit of taking muscle relaxants only provides short-term relief.

Cyclobenzaprine (Flexeril) is a recommended medication for muscle spasms and for providing relief from muscle pain.

Anticonvulsants:

The main purpose of these medications is to treat seizure disorders. However, they have been found to be effective in reducing pain in fibromyalgia sufferers. They work by treating any discomfort in the nervous system. Here are a few examples of anticonvulsants used to treat people suffering from fibromyalgia: Gabapentin (Gralise), Lamotrigine (Lamictal), Pregabalin (Lyrica) and Topiramate (Topamax).

Anti-Anxieties:

As many fibromyalgia sufferers suffer from anxiety which has the effect of increasing pain, muscular tension and mood disorders, anti-anxiety medications can play an important role. An anxious state of mind is also intimately linked to disturbed sleep patterns and depression. By relieving anxiety, pain can often be reduced, mood enhanced and muscle tension reduced. Examples of anti-anxiety medications include Diazepam (Valium) and Alprazolam Niravam). If a fibromyalgia sufferer has restless legs at night, then, Clonazepam (Klonopin) may be prescribed.

Corticosteroids:

as fibromyalgia is not an inflammatory condition, corticosteroid medications provide no benefit whatsoever in treating the symptoms.

This list of medications is not all inclusive, but is just given as an example of what may be prescribed for your condition. Your physician will be able to prescribe a treatment program that is suitable for your condition, based on the diagnosis that has been undertaken.

Various other treatments should be incorporated as part of a treatment program. These include: counseling, cognitive behavior therapy to help the individual feel good about themselves and to help them deal with stressful situations. This therapy is useful as a stressful condition can increase the pain perception with the result that it can aggravate the symptoms.

Chapter 9. Alternative Treatments

Many alternative treatments are available which can provide relief for individuals who suffer from fibromyalgia. The following is a list of treatments which have proved to be beneficial.

Chiropractor:

A qualified chiropractor will be able to provide relieve for neck pain, shoulder pain, headaches and muscular pain through a process of motions which are applied to pressure points on the body. The practitioner accomplishes this by means of stretching, gentle pressure and thrusts by using hand adjustments. All of this may prove beneficial to help reduce pain and increase quality of life.

Massage Therapy:

A good massage therapist who is fully trained, using a Swedish massage technique and the application of oil will stimulate the circulation and metabolism. A Swedish massage works on the superficial layers of the muscle and is combined with joint movements.

Applying pressure with friction, together with stroking and kneading the muscles has the effect of returning the blood flow back to the heart. If a more aggressive form of massage therapy is used, this involves stimulating tissue layers and is accomplished by applying firmer pressure to these areas. The therapist will use thumbs and/or elbows which can apply greater force which has the effect of reducing tension in the patient.

Neuromuscular Massage:

This is similar to acupressure and shiatsu and is another form of deep tissue massage which is designed to target pain areas.

Biofeedback:

This is a technique where electronics are used to help relax the mind and body. This treatment has been shown to assist with chronic pain conditions such as fibromyalgia. Sensors are used to analyze various processes of the body such as: breathing, heart rate, sweat production, the temperature of the body and tension of the muscles.

Homeopathic Medicine:

This is a treatment process where diluted substances which can be of animal, mineral or plant origin are used to help reduce pain.

Herbal Medication:

I have discussed the use of herbs elsewhere in this book. They can be very effective at increasing energy levels and normalizing sleep patterns.

Acupuncture:

Acupuncture is a process where needles are inserted under the skin at various pressure points. The practitioner manipulates the needles and as a result endorphins (a hormone compound that is manufactured by the body in response to pain or extreme physical exertion) are released into the bloodstream. One of the purposes of acupuncture is to increase energy flow by removing energy blocks in the energy channels. Research has shown that this form of treatment can change the actions of chemistry in the brain. Acupuncture can help reduce pain for prolonged periods of time.

Electro Acupuncture:

In this form of treatment needles are also used but they are connected to wires that release small amounts of electrical current. Other forms of therapy can also be used in combination with electro acupuncture during this treatment.

Meditation:

This treatment method relaxes the body and puts it in a peaceful state of mind. The purpose of this treatment is to focus your mind on releasing any stress factors in your life and to only concentrate on positive aspects which will enhance your quality of life.

All the above alternative treatments have their merits, however, before deciding on a particular alternative treatment it is best to discuss this with your physician, as they may have some suggestions as to which treatment may prove most beneficial, taking into account any medications which you may have been prescribed for your condition.

Chapter 10. Nutrition

Eating a healthy well-balanced diet is necessary for all individuals, whether they suffer from fibromyalgia or not. The body needs adequate amounts of various vitamins, minerals, fiber and essential fatty acids which are contained within various food groups as well as protein, carbohydrates, fats and starches. If the diet is lacking in these essential nutrients, then it might be advisable to implement a vitamin and mineral supplementation program.

Those individuals who suffer from fibromyalgia have found that certain types of food will aggravate symptoms of the illness. The following is a list of some of the food types that have been identified as causing problems for fibromyalgia sufferers:

- Foods that are high in saturated fats which include fried foods and a lot of the junk foods.

- Foods that are high in calories

- Foods that contain preservatives, coloring and have a high salt content.

- Foods that contain NutraSweet (aspartame), saccharine and monosodium glutamate (MSG). Some of these ingredients have been identified as stimulating pain receptor sites located in the spinal cord.

- Certain red meats such as salt cured bacon.

- Dairy foods that contain high amounts of fat.

- White sugar and white flour. Interestingly refining sugar and flour removes a lot of the trace minerals which are required in minute amounts by the body to perform its many functions, as well as the fiber content in the flour.

- Alcohol.

- Chocolate and other foods which have a high sugar content.

- Coffee and tea containing caffeine.

- Carbonated drinks.

- Tobacco products.

As mentioned above, pursuing good eating habits can improve the overall health of the body. Some guidelines to consider include:

- Elevating serotonin levels. Serotonin is a neurotransmitter which is involved in many functions of the brain such as pain perception, regulating sleep patterns and providing a general feeling of well-being. Carbohydrate foods can help raise serotonin levels especially if they are taken during the daytime; complex carbohydrates such as grains, beans and other starchy foods; as well as dark chocolate (but only take small amounts) can all prove beneficial.

- An adequate supply of protein is important. Some researchers theorize that some of the abnormalities in the tissue which are linked to fibromyalgia may be due to a lack of sufficient protein in the diet. In addition, eating recommended daily levels of protein has been associated with reduced levels of pain and stiffness. One thing to bear in mind is that an excessive consumption of red meat can lead to an inflammatory condition in the body; therefore white meat can be more preferable as well as oily fish which contain the essential fatty acid omega-3. Soy protein is another good source of protein, and the advantage of this is that it is virtually fat-free and does not cause an inflammatory condition in the body.

- Some people find that avoiding drinking fluids with meals helps to relieve some of the symptoms of the condition.

- It helps to keep your body hydrated during the day, this can be accomplished by drinking plenty of water—at least eight glasses. Try not to drink tap water if possible as this contains various chemicals which are added by the water company. A far better source of water is to use either filtered water or still bottled water—not carbonated water.

- Try to avoid being in direct sunlight for long periods of time. However, sunlight is important for the synthesis of vitamin D in the body. Therefore, it might be wise to add a vitamin D supplement to your diet.

It might be that a little experimentation is required to determine which foods trigger symptoms and which don't. It is best to just remove one food type at a time, and if this particular food triggers symptoms, then that is one to remove from the diet. On the other hand, if it does not cause any problems then it can be added back into the diet and then another food can be selected for removal. If several foods are removed at the same time, then it is difficult to identify which one is the culprit.

Being able to identify a selection of foods which do not trigger symptoms will ensure that energy levels are maintained and this will help to maintain a feeling of well-being. It may be a little time-consuming doing all this food research, but the end result will be well worth the effort.

Chapter 11. Herbs and Supplements

Various initial studies show that some medicinal herbs and natural supplements can help treat symptoms of fibromyalgia.

Many people therefore take herbs and vitamin supplements in conjunction with alternative therapies. Magnesium and malic acid when taken together may help reduce pain. Studies show that individuals who suffer from fibromyalgia often have low levels of magnesium and malic acid. Gotu Kola which is used in traditional Chinese and Indian medicine may provide some relief from anxiety. I have provided a list of herbs and supplements below for you to consider.

However it is important that you discuss any proposed supplement program with your physician before commencing, as some herbal supplements may react against medications which you may be taking.

5 HTP:

5-HTP (5-Hydroxytryptophan) is produced in the body from one of the essential amino acids called tryptophan. 5-HTP is a precursor for the neurotransmitter serotonin and the hormone melatonin.

Serotonin is converted into melatonin which is needed for the regulation of waking and sleeping cycles. By increasing serotonin levels, melatonin levels will also increase which will help normalize sleep patterns.

Serotonin is therefore intimately linked to fibromyalgia pain and it is also linked to depression and sleep patterns.

5-HTP works by increasing the levels of serotonin in the brain. Researchers theorize that it works by reducing the number of tender points in individuals who suffer from fibromyalgia. It accomplishes this by affecting systems that control pain in the brain stem.

In one double-blind, placebo controlled study 50 individuals who suffered from fibromyalgia were either given 5-HTP or a placebo. Four weeks later, those taking 5-HTP experienced a major reduction in pain as well as the number of tender points, anxiety, fatigue, stiffness and improved sleep patterns. They experienced only mild side effects.

Also, in a study published in the journal Alternative Medicine Review, researchers stated that fibromyalgia sufferers who supplemented with 5-HTP would not only improve their fibromyalgia pains, but would also improve symptoms of anxiety, depression and insomnia.

5-HTP is obtained from the seeds of the plant Griffonia Simplicifolia—which grows in Africa. It is manufactured into a pill form which can be obtained from health food stores, on the Internet, and at various drug stores.

Individuals take 5-HTP for a variety of conditions including:
- Anxiety
- Depression
- Fibromyalgia
- Insomnia
- Migraine
- Weight-loss

Melatonin:

Melatonin is a hormone whose precursor is serotonin. It is readily available as an over-the-counter (OTC) supplement in health food stores, on the Internet and in some drugstores. It is often taken to cause drowsiness and enhance sleep patterns. Preliminary studies show that melatonin can be an effective treatment for fibromyalgia pain. The majority of people with fibromyalgia experience disturbed sleep patterns, and this is one supplement that can prove really helpful.

Gotu Kola:

Used extensively in Indian Ayurvedic and Traditional Chinese Medicine (TCM), gotu kola exhibits anti-inflammatory effects as well as increasing blood flow throughout the entire body. It does this by strengthening veins and capillaries. Gotu kola is also used to treat connective tissue disorders, excess fatigue, disturbed sleep patterns, and depression.

MSM (Methylsulfonylmethane):

A natural sulfur compound used to treat pain in joints and connective tissue.

Olive Leaf:

Well known for helping to boost a weakened immune system. In individuals who have been diagnosed with fibromyalgia, they reported increased energy levels, improvements in mood and a better sense of purpose in life.

St John's Wort:

St. John's Wort has not proved helpful in treating fibromyalgia. Its main use is in the treatment of mild to moderate depression, where it has proved to be as effective as Selective Serotonin Reuptake Inhibitors (SSRIs), such as Prozac or Zoloft. Depression is often associated with fibromyalgia. St. John's Wort has also been used for the relief of menopause, hot flashes and night sweats.

Care should be taken if you are taking antidepressants, especially monoamine oxidase (MAO) inhibitors. It is best to consult your doctor before commencing taking St. John's Wort.

S-adenosylmethionine (SAMe):

S-adenosylmethionine (SAMe) is a compound that is made from the essential amino acid methionine via the homocysteine pathway. It is required to support the functions of the immune system as well as cell membranes.

It is involved in making and breaking down certain neurotransmitters including serotonin, norepinephrine, and dopamine. It also plays a key role in the formation of cartilage and genetic material (DNA).

Various studies have been conducted suggesting SAMe may be of benefit to individuals suffering from fibromyalgia. In one such double-blind study, 44 individuals suffering from fibromyalgia were given 800 mg of SAMe or a placebo each day. After a six weeks period there were major improvements in pain, mood, fatigue and muscle stiffness as well as improved sleep patterns in the group taking SAMe.

There are some cautions with regard to people taking SAMe. Individuals with bipolar disorder should avoid SAMe as it may make manic attacks worse. Also, anyone taking the medication levodopa which is prescribed for Parkinson's disease should also avoid taking SAMe. Individuals who take any form of antidepressants should not take SAMe without first discussing this with their doctor. The safety aspect of taking SAMe by children or pregnant or nursing women has not been determined.

Magnesium:

Magnesium is a mineral that occurs naturally in such foods as green leafy vegetables, nuts, seeds and whole grains. It is also available as a stand-alone supplement; and is also often combined with calcium to form a calcium magnesium supplement. Vitamin D is needed for the efficient uptake by the body of these minerals.

Magnesium is important as it is needed for more than 300 biochemical reactions in the body. When magnesium is combined with malic acid (a fruit acid which occurs naturally in apples) it has proved beneficial for people suffering from fibromyalgia. Research shows that sufferers often have low levels of magnesium and malic acid. Both of these are needed for the production of adenosine triphosphate (ATP) which is needed for the generation of energy in body cells.

Several studies have been undertaken using a magnesium/malic acid combination. One double-blind study involved 24 people with fibromyalgia to determine the effectiveness of this combination: (magnesium 50 mg three times a day and malic acid 200 milligrams three times a day). After a period of four-week participants gained no more benefit than the group who were taking a placebo.

Following this disappointing start, the participants were then put on a larger dose of the combination for a period of six months (magnesium 300 mg a day and malic acid 1200 mg a day). At the end of the trial period, this increased dose and timeline produced a significant improvement in the pain threshold and tenderness points.

Vitamin D:

Vitamin D is needed by the body for the efficient uptake of calcium and magnesium. It is often thought that vitamin D is synthesized in the body by the actions of sunlight. However, in areas of the world where there is insufficient sunlight, then a vitamin D deficiency can occur.

Also, when individuals go on vacation, the actions of applying a high factor sunscreen also preclude the body from synthesizing vitamin D by the actions of sunlight.

Researchers have determined that aches and pains which do not meet the requirements for a diagnosis of fibromyalgia are often due to a lack of vitamin D.

One study published in the Mayo Clinic proceedings examined 150 people with non-specific musculoskeletal pain. Researchers found that 93 percent of these individuals were deficient in vitamin D.

In a different study, the levels of vitamin D were assessed in 75 individuals who fell within the criteria determined by the American College of rheumatology for a diagnosis of fibromyalgia. Although no relationship was established between vitamin D levels and musculoskeletal symptoms, a vitamin D deficiency was implicated in anxiety and depression levels in individuals with fibromyalgia.

Vitamin B12:
A study in Sweden identified low levels of vitamin B12 (Cyanocobalamin) in the cerebrospinal fluid of individuals with fibromyalgia as well as those individuals suffering from chronic fatigue syndrome (CFS).

The study group comprised 12 women who had been diagnosed with fibromyalgia, in addition to 18 healthy women.

Homocysteine (a type of protein formed from the essential amino acid methionine) levels in the cerebrospinal fluid were more than three times higher in the 12 women with fibromyalgia, when compared to the 18 healthy women. The levels of vitamin B12 were significantly low in the cerebrospinal fluid in 7 out of 12 people with fibromyalgia.

Capsaicin Cream:
Capsaicin is one of the main active ingredients in chili peppers. One of the main benefits is that it is used as a temporary relief from pain.

When it is applied to the skin, capsaicin cream depletes substance P—a neurochemical that is involved in pain transmission. Individuals who have been diagnosed with fibromyalgia have higher levels of substance P.

One study determined the effectiveness of capsaicin in fibromyalgia sufferers. Participants applied 0.025 percent capsaicin cream four times a day to tender points. Four weeks later they experienced reduced pain.

A good dose to start with is 0.025 percent capsaicin cream applied four times a day (which is in line with the above study), should this dose prove ineffective then a 0.075 percent concentration can be used under the direction of a healthcare practitioner. Capsaicin cream should be applied directly to areas of joint or muscle pain or itching.

One possible side effect is that the cream can cause a burning or stinging sensation to the area where it has been applied. Not everyone experiences this side effect, and the fact that someone does not have this experience, does not mean that the cream is not working. Many practitioners recommend that the cream should be applied for a period of four consecutive weeks so that a proper evaluation of its effectiveness can be determined.

In addition to being used for fibromyalgia pain, other uses include:

- Back pain
- Bursitis
- Joint pain
- Muscle pain
- Nerve Pain
- Osteoarthritis
- Post-herpetic neuralgia
- Post-surgical neuropathic pain
- Pruritus (itching)
- Rheumatoid arthritis

Capsaicin cream can be obtained from health food stores, on the Internet or from some drug stores.

L-Carnitine:

L-Carnitine is a non-essential amino acid which is formed in the body from the essential amino acid lysine. Some studies suggest that l-carnitine provides pain relief for individuals who suffer from fibromyalgia. In one particular study participants who took l-carnitine had greater improvements in pain relief than those participants who took a placebo.

L-carnitine can be obtained in supplement form from health food stores, on the Internet and in some drug stores.

Probiotics:

Probiotics are available in capsule forms that contain beneficial bacteria needed by the gut to ensure good health. Friendly bacterial is needed for the final breakdown and absorption of food as well as to keep unfriendly bacteria and yeasts at bay.

Probiotics also assist with digestive problems often associated with irritable bowel syndrome—which is one of the symptoms associated with fibromyalgia.

And finally, individuals have claimed that the following herbs have helped them manage their fibromyalgia symptoms:

Black Cohosh:

A member of the buttercup family – taken for hot flashes and menopausal problems

Cayenne:

Improves the circulatory system

Echinacea:

Provides support to the immune system

Lavender:

A member of the mint family – used to reduce nervous tension and relieve pain

Milk Thistle:

Provides a detoxifying and support function for the liver.

Chapter 12. Exercise

Mild to moderate exercise has been proven to be beneficial for fibromyalgia sufferers, as it helps reduce the perception of pain. While it may be thought that exercise may be detrimental, exactly the opposite has proved to be the case.

If done correctly exercise will reduce the deconditioning effect which is the result of the fibromyalgia symptoms. Deconditioning means that muscles as well as the heart lose their ability to function properly or to put it another way "be in good shape". This being out of shape may result in an increased risk of trauma to the muscle area as a result of no exercises being undertaken.

Interestingly, many people who suffer from fibromyalgia will experience symptoms that are worse on one side of the body as opposed to the other side. This has the effect of reducing motion on one side of the body which may affect posture and increase pain.

An exercise program will increase the ability of the circulatory system to perform its function more effectively. This can lead to an improved mental outlook which has the effect of assisting the body during stressful times in a person's life.

It is best that an individual starts with non-stressful stretching exercises after getting warmed up. These exercises should be slow, without any vigorous stretching of the muscles. The whole purpose of the exercise is to help keep the muscles loose and improve the motion range of the joints and muscles.

Exercises should also be of a low-impact variety. Good exercises to consider include: walking, swimming or bike riding. Many people find that adding a 30 minutes exercise program into their daily life can be accomplished without compromising any other activities of the day.

You may have heard the saying "no pain no gain". Well, this should not be heeded with someone who is suffering from fibromyalgia. Excessive pain may indicate that your exercise program has been too vigorous and as a result a muscle group may have been damaged. If this is the case, then it is important to rest so that the muscles can repair themselves.

For an exercise program to be most effective it should be done on a regular basis. It is important to do exercises that you enjoy doing; if exercise is regarded as a daily chore then it is only a matter of time before it is discontinued. The benefits of doing daily exercises can include better sleep patterns and reduced pain.

It is also important to monitor progress and also monitor symptoms of the syndrome. If you feel any soreness in your muscles or there is a flare-up in your symptoms, then it is highly likely that the exercises you are doing may be unsuitable for you and a more gentle exercise regime may be more beneficial.

Chapter 13. Rehabilitation and Coping

One of the main purposes of a rehabilitation program is to help an individual formulate different strategies to cope with their condition and at the same time, improve their quality of life. Coping strategies should be formulated by using a professional with experience in helping people who suffer from chronic pain and daily discomfort which affects their daily routine. Team members such as counselors, psychologists and social workers can help an individual to formulate strategies to assist them at work and with other aspects of their daily life.

I am sure that you have heard of the saying that "knowledge is power". Therefore, one of the ways a person can help themselves cope with the syndrome is to do as much research as possible into the symptoms and treatments available.

A lack of understanding of the nature of muscle pain or where the trigger pain points are will make it difficult for a person to structure their day in such a way as to alleviate any situation which may cause an increase in pain, and also make it more difficult to protect the body against any further injury.

It is usual to have really good days when the symptoms are bearable, and then some really bad days when the symptoms seem unbearable.

When you have good days, it is a good idea to make a list of family and friends you can contact for help when you have bad days.

The following is a list of some things that you can do to provide a level of relief from the symptoms of this condition.

Medication:
It is important to take the medication prescribed by your physician in the recommended amount which will help you deal with the pain and depressive symptoms which is associated with this condition.

Nutrition:
It is important to get adequate nutrition to fulfil your body's requirements. This is especially important for a person who has food sensitivities. Adequate nutrition can be obtained by eating a balanced diet. However, if there are shortfalls in your diet then a

supplementation program using vitamins, minerals, essential fatty acids and fiber may prove helpful.

Sleep:

Disturbed sleep patterns are one of the conditions associated with fibromyalgia. It is important to make sure that your bedroom is as dark as possible, and that the bed is warm to prevent any pain triggers such as muscle spasms. Consider taking a warm bath or shower before going to bed as this will help to promote sleep. Also, a cup of warm milk before going to bed might also prove relaxing and help you sleep. Finally make sure your bed is comfortable and use extra pillows and blankets if necessary.

Have a Positive Mental Attitude:

Depression is one of the symptoms brought on by fibromyalgia. In addition to taking antidepressants, it is also important to surround yourself with positive people and avoid negative ones at all costs. Although there are times throughout life when worries come to the fore, it is important to put these situations into perspective and try to maintain a positive balance in your life as much as possible.

Massage Therapy:

Some researchers feel that fibromyalgia is induced by excess lactic acid. In a patient with fibromyalgia, approximately 18 tender areas on the body, when touched, generate a shooting pain which transmits throughout the body. Massage therapy has been shown to soothe these areas by releasing the build-up of any lactic acid. Although touching these areas as mentioned can be painful, a massage can be very effective at reducing pain in the sensitive areas.

Alternative Therapies:

Several alternative therapies can be considered as mentioned elsewhere in this book. Many of these alternative therapies have proved highly beneficial for someone who is suffering from fibromyalgia.

Exercise:

Exercise can be very beneficial for anyone suffering from fibromyalgia. However, it is best to start with a gentle exercise program and increase the exercises as appropriate. Swimming is a very effective exercise treatment for anyone who suffers from pain when they move their limbs.

Having a daily exercise routine can be beneficial for reducing anxiety and stress which has the added benefit of helping you to sleep better and decrease pain.

A physical therapist should be consulted to design an appropriate exercise program. Remember each person is different and different exercise strategies may be required to stimulate the interest of the individual to take into account such things as where the individual pain trigger points are, as well as their overall level of fitness.

It is important to enjoy whatever exercise program is chosen; otherwise it becomes a chore with a likely prospect that the exercise program will be discontinued.

Deep Breathing Exercises:

In addition to taking medication, try to do some deep breathing exercises which will help to reduce anxiety and stress.

Support groups:

And networking can be highly beneficial as part of a rehabilitation program. Psychologists know that individuals who suffer from a variety of illnesses or diseases who involve themselves in support groups containing people with a similar condition to themselves most often fair better emotionally and psychologically than those who do not attend support group sessions. A good starting point is to ask at your local hospital or clinic for contact details of support groups and/or networking organizations in your area.

If you do not feel comfortable being part of a support group, then consider talking directly with an individual one-on-one who has similar symptoms to yourself. It is often reassuring to know that it is not just you who has the condition, but other people suffer just as much too.

How to contact individuals? Often social workers and physicians will have contact details of individuals who are prepared to share their individual experiences with other sufferers. All you need to do is ask.

People who suffer from fibromyalgia should be their own best advocate—and the best way to do this is to participate in a rehabilitation program designed specifically for people who suffer from this condition. Researching as much as you can about fibromyalgia, and learning from others in a similar situation to yourself, as well as implementing a regular exercise program is all part of an effective rehabilitation and coping program.

It is impossible for anyone who is suffering from fibromyalgia to totally eradicate all the symptoms of their condition. However, they can learn to cope with the condition by following some of the strategies mentioned above. It is also a good idea to discuss these coping strategies with your physician and ask if there are any other strategies that he/she might want to add to this list.

About The Author

Brian B Jacques started in business at a young age, and over the ensuing years, he has developed several very successful businesses. But his main interest for the past 40 years has been in natural health research and publishing.

Brian has presented seminars worldwide on such diverse subjects as Health Related issues, Motivation and Personal Development. In addition he has written numerous books, newsletters and articles on these subjects.

His very popular series of Mini Health Books has circulated widely around the world, and many more titles are in preparation.

Brian is a highly motivated individual, so much so that in 1985 he received a UK Industrial Society award for his work in the Motivation and Personal Development fields.

Brian has the following mottos:

- If something does not work out for you, then don't give up, but keep trying, trying, trying until finally you succeed.

- Success or failure in any endeavor is in your own hands.

Brian and his wife divide their time between East Yorkshire, UK and Florida, USA.

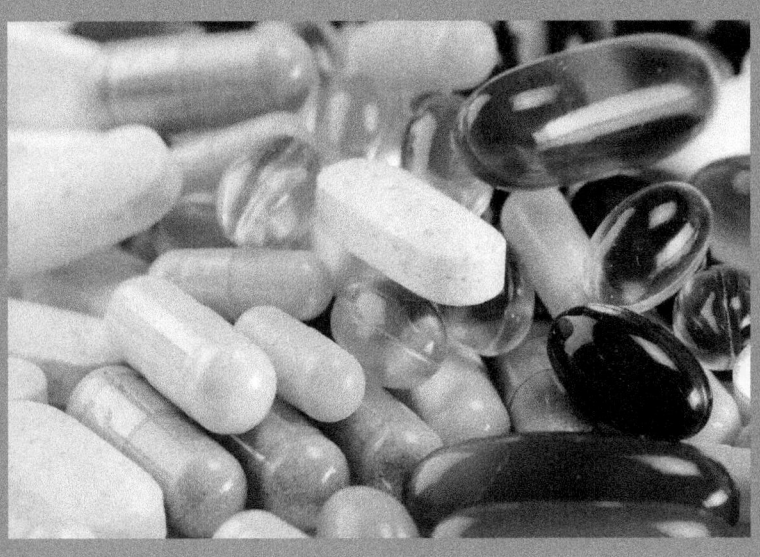

www.ingramcontent.com/pod-product-compliance
Lightning Source LLC
Chambersburg PA
CBHW071250280526
45788CB00004B/1663